**Combined Med Peds Residency Match
Selection Criteria and Programs Requirements**

By

**Match A Doc
and
Residency Guide**

Contents

Introduction

Combined Medicine/Pediatrics Residency Match Selection Criteria and Programs Requirements

A must-read book for residency applicants.

This book is the must-read book and most single important piece you buy in your battle for residency. This is the Combined Med Peds Residency Match Selection Criteria and Programs Requirements book (Combined Medicine Pediatrics Residency or Combined Med/Peds Residency) that contains up-to-date information about all the programs in the United States for both AMGs and IMGs. Why this book is essential to match? It has been shown that applying to programs that you don't match their minimum criteria is just waste of money and time. It is very important that you apply to those programs that you meet their requirements and this why we decided to make your life easier by gathering the information you need in one book. The information was gathered from program directors, coordinators, chiefs, faculty and residents. It includes Programs names, Programs codes, States, Addresses, Phones, Faxes, Percentage of IMGs in the programs, Minimum USMLE Step 1 and Step 2 Score Requirements, Attempts on any step, CS requirement at time of application, USCE Requirements, Cut-Off time since graduation, Programs offering couple match and Visas Sponsored or accepted. We have more than 10 years experience in the match field and our book is the proof that will help you to get the highest number of interviews to increase your chances in the match journey.

Alabama

University of Alabama Medical Center Combined Med-Peds Residency Program

Specialty: Combined Internal Medicine/Pediatrics
Program name: University of Alabama Medical Center Program
Program code: 700-01-32-115
NRMP Code: 1007700C0
Program type: University-based
State: Alabama
Address: Children's Hospital Alabama, Building ACC604,
        1600 7th Ave S, Birmingham, AL 35233-0011
Phone: (205) 934-5004
Fax: (205) 638-9589
Percentage of IMGs in the program: 0%
Minimum USMLE Step 1 Score Requirement: No limits set

Minimum USMLE Step 2 Score Requirement: No limits set
Attempts on any step: No limits set
CS required at time of application: No
USCE Requirement: None
Cut-Off time since graduation: 10 years
Program offers couple match: Yes
Visas Sponsored or accepted: J1 visa and H1b visa

University of South Alabama Combined Med-Peds Residency Program

Specialty: Combined Internal Medicine-Pediatrics
Program name: University of South Alabama Program
Program code: 700-01-32-085
NRMP Code: 1852700C0
Program type: University-based
State: Alabama
Address: USA Children's and Women's Hospital, Medicine-Pediatrics Program,
          1700 Center St, Mobile, AL 36604
Phone: (251) 415-1087
Fax: (251) 415-1087
Percentage of IMGs in the program: 0%

Minimum USMLE Step 1 Score Requirement: 205
Minimum USMLE Step 2 Score Requirement: 205
Attempts on any step: No limits set
CS required at time of application: No
USCE Requirement: None
Cut-Off time since graduation: No limits set
Program offers couple match: Yes
Visas Sponsored or accepted: J1 visa

Arizona

Banner Good Samaritan Medical Center Combined Med-Peds Residency Program

Specialty: Combined Internal Medicine-Pediatrics
Program name: Banner Good Samaritan Medical Center Program
Program code: 700-03-14-001
NRMP Code: 1011700C0
Program type: Community-based university affiliated hospital
State: Arizona
Address: Banner Good Samaritan Med Center, Department of Medicine,

1111 E McDowell Rd, Phoenix, AZ 85006
Phone: (602) 839-3644
Fax: (602) 839-2084
Percentage of IMGs in the program: 0%
Minimum USMLE Step 1 Score Requirement: 200
Minimum USMLE Step 2 Score Requirement: 210
Attempts on any step: No limits set
CS required at time of application: Yes
USCE Requirement: Yes
Cut-Off time since graduation: 2 years
Program offers couple match: Yes
Visas Sponsored or accepted: No visa

Arkansas

University of Arkansas for Medical Sciences Combined Internal Med-Peds Residency Program

Specialty: Combined Internal Medicine-Pediatrics
Program name: University of Arkansas for Medical Sciences Program
Program code: 700-04-14-002

NRMP Code: 1018700C0
Program type: University-based
State: Arkansas
Address: University of Arkansas for Med Sciences, Internal Med H/S Office #634,
           4301 W Markham St, Little Rock, AR 72205-7199
Phone: (501) 686-5162
Fax: (501) 686-6001
Percentage of IMGs in the program: 25%
Minimum USMLE Step 1 Score Requirement: 210
Minimum USMLE Step 2 Score Requirement: 220
Attempts on any step: No limits set
CS required at time of application: Yes as well as ECFMG certificate
USCE Requirement: None
Cut-Off time since graduation: 7 years
Program offers couple match: Yes
Visas Sponsored or accepted: J1 visa and H1b visa

California

University of California (San Diego) Combined Med-Peds Residency Program

Specialty: Combined Internal Medicine-Pediatrics
Program name: University of California (San Diego) Program
Program code: 700-05-14-099
Program type: University-based
State: California
Address: UCSD Medical Center, Combined Med/Peds #8425,
            200 W Arbor Dr, San Diego, CA 92103-8425
Phone: (619) 471-0434
Fax: (619) 543-6529
Percentage of IMGs in the program: 0%
Minimum USMLE Step 1 Score Requirement: No limits set
Minimum USMLE Step 2 Score Requirement: No limits set
Attempts on any step: Must pass on first attempt
CS required at time of application: No but PTAL required
USCE Requirement: None
Cut-Off time since graduation: 5 years
Program offers couple match: Yes
Visas Sponsored or accepted: J1 visa

UCLA Medical Center Combined Med-Peds Residency Program

Specialty: Combined Internal Medicine/Pediatrics
Program name: UCLA Medical Center Program
Program code: 700-05-32-130
Program type: University-based
State: California
Address: Ronald Reagan UCLA Medical Center, Suite 7501,

757 Westwood Plaza, Los Angeles, CA 90095-7417
Phone: (310) 267 9648
Percentage of IMGs in the program: 0%
Minimum USMLE Step 1 Score Requirement: 220
Minimum USMLE Step 2 Score Requirement: 220
Attempts on any step: Must pass on first attempt
CS required at time of application: No
USCE Requirement: Yes
Cut-Off time since graduation: No limits set
Program offers couple match: Yes
Visas Sponsored or accepted: No visa

University of Southern California/LAC USC Medical Center Combined Med/Peds Residency Program

Specialty: Combined Internal Medicine-Pediatrics
Program name: University of Southern California/LAC+USC Medical Center Program
Program code: 700-05-32-005
NRMP Code: 1033700C0
Program type: University-based
State: California
Address: LAC+USC Medical Center, Combined IM/Pediatrics Suite 115,
          2020 Zonal Ave, Los Angeles, CA 90033-1084
Phone: (323) 226-5700
Fax: (323) 226-3853
Percentage of IMGs in the program: 0%
Minimum USMLE Step 1 Score Requirement: No limits set
Minimum USMLE Step 2 Score Requirement: No limits set
Attempts on any step: No limits set
CS required at time of application: Yes including ECFMG certificate and PTAL
USCE Requirement: None
Cut-Off time since graduation: No limits set
Program offers couple match: Yes

Visas Sponsored or accepted: J1 visa

Loma Linda University Combined Med-Peds Residency Program

Specialty: Combined Internal Medicine/Pediatrics
Program name: Loma Linda University Program
Program code: 700-05-32-003
NRMP Code: 1024700C0
Program type: University-based
State: California
Address: Loma Linda University Medical Center, Coleman Pavilion A1111,
          11175 Campus St, Loma Linda, CA 92350
Phone: (909) 558-4174
Fax: (909) 558-4184
Percentage of IMGs in the program: 0%
Minimum USMLE Step 1 Score Requirement: 200
Minimum USMLE Step 2 Score Requirement: 205
Attempts on any step: Must pass on first attempt
CS required at time of application: Yes as well as ECFMG Certificate and PTAL.
USCE Requirement: None
Cut-Off time since graduation: 5 years
Program offers couple match: No

Visas Sponsored or accepted: J1 visa

Colorado

University of Colorado School of Medicine Combined Med-Peds Residency Program

Specialty: Combined Internal Medicine/Pediatrics
Program name: University of Colorado School of Medicine Program
Program code: 700-07-00-001
NRMP Code: 1076700CO
Program type: University-based
State: Colorado
Address: University of Colorado School of Medicine, Academic Office One Box B177,
          12631 E 17th Ave, Aurora, CO 80045
Phone: (303) 724-6595
Fax: (303) 724-1799
Percentage of IMGs in the program: 0%
Minimum USMLE Step 1 Score Requirement: No limits set
Minimum USMLE Step 2 Score Requirement: No limits set
Attempts on any step: No limits set
CS required at time of application: No

USCE Requirement: Yes 4 months
Cut-Off time since graduation: 2 years
Program offers couple match: Yes
Visas Sponsored or accepted: No visa

Connecticut

Yale-New Haven Medical Center (Waterbury) Combined Med-Peds Residency Program

Specialty: Combined Internal Medicine/Pediatrics
Program name: Yale-New Haven Medical Center (Waterbury) Program
Program code: 700-08-14-127
NRMP Code: 1089700C0
Program type: University-based
State: Connecticut
Address: Yale University School of Medicine, PO Box 208086,
        333 Cedar St, New Haven, CT 06520-8086
Phone: (203) 785-7941
Fax: 203-785-3922
Percentage of IMGs in the program: 0%
Minimum USMLE Step 1 Score Requirement: No limits set

Minimum USMLE Step 2 Score Requirement: No limits set
Attempts on any step: Must pass on first attempt
CS required at time of application: Yes
USCE Requirement: Yes 2 months
Cut-Off time since graduation: No limits set
Program offers couple match: Yes
Visas Sponsored or accepted: J1 visa and H1b visa

Delaware

Jefferson Medical College/Christiana Care Health Services Combined Med-Peds Residency Program

Specialty: Combined Internal Medicine/Pediatrics
Program name: Jefferson Medical College/Christiana Care Health Services Program
Program code: 700-09-14-009
NRMP Code: 1099700C0

Program type: Community-based university affiliated hospital
State: Delaware
Address: Christiana Care Health System, PO Box 6001 Suite 2E70,
            4755 Ogletown-Stanton Rd, Newark, DE 19718
Phone: (302) 733-2313
Fax: (302) 733-4339
Percentage of IMGs in the program: 0%
Minimum USMLE Step 1 Score Requirement: No limits set
Minimum USMLE Step 2 Score Requirement: No limits set
Attempts on any step: No limits set
CS required at time of application: No
USCE Requirement: None
Cut-Off time since graduation: No limits set
Program offers couple match: Yes
Visas Sponsored or accepted: J1 visa

District of Columbia

Georgetown University Hospital Combined Med-Peds Residency Program

Specialty: Combined Internal Medicine/Pediatrics
Program name: Georgetown University Hospital Program
Program code: 700-10-14-129
NRMP Code: 1801700C0
Program type: University-based
State: District of Columbia
Address: Georgetown University Hospital, 5 PHC,

3800 Reservoir Rd NW, Washington, DC 20007-2197
Phone: (202) 444-8492
Fax: (202) 444-7797
Percentage of IMGs in the program: 0%
Minimum USMLE Step 1 Score Requirement: 220
Minimum USMLE Step 2 Score Requirement: 220
Attempts on any step: No limits set
CS required at time of application: No
USCE Requirement: Yes
Cut-Off time since graduation: No limits set
Program offers couple match: Yes
Visas Sponsored or accepted: J1 visa

Florida

University of South Florida Morsani Combined Med/Peds Residency Program

Specialty: Combined Internal Medicine/Pediatrics
Program name: University of South Florida Morsani Program
Program code: 700-11-32-125
NRMP Code: 1109700C0
Program type: University-based
State: Florida
Address: University of South Florida College of Medicine, 5th Floor STC Room 5036,
          2 Tampa General Circle, Tampa, FL 33606
Phone: (813) 259-8725
Fax: (813) 259-8792
Percentage of IMGs in the program: 15%
Minimum USMLE Step 1 Score Requirement: No limits set
Minimum USMLE Step 2 Score Requirement: No limits set
Attempts on any step: Maximum of two attempts one each step
CS required at time of application: No
USCE Requirement: None
Cut-Off time since graduation: 5 years
Program offers couple match: Yes

Visas Sponsored or accepted: J1 visa

Jackson Memorial Hospital/Jackson Health System Combined Med/Peds Residency Program

Specialty: Combined Internal Medicine/Pediatrics
Program name: Jackson Memorial Hospital/Jackson Health System Program
Program code: 700-11-14-086
NRMP Code: 1104700C0
Program type: University-based
State: Florida
Address: University of Miami/Jackson Memorial Hospital, Central 600D,
          1611 NW 12th Ave, Miami, FL 33136
Phone: (305) 585-5954
Fax: (305) 585-7381
Percentage of IMGs in the program: 0%
Minimum USMLE Step 1 Score Requirement: No limits set
Minimum USMLE Step 2 Score Requirement: No limits set
Attempts on any step: Must pass on first attempt
CS required at time of application: No
USCE Requirement: Yes 5 months
Cut-Off time since graduation: 5 years
Program offers couple match: Yes

Visas Sponsored or accepted: J1 visa

Illinois

University of Illinois College of Medicine at Peoria Combined Med-Peds Residency Program

Specialty: Combined Internal Medicine/Pediatrics
Program name: University of Illinois College of Medicine at Peoria Program
Program code: 700-16-32-015
NRMP Code: 1175700C0
Program type: Community-based university affiliated hospital
State: Illinois
Address: OSF St Francis Medical Center, Med/Peds Program,
        530 NE Glen Oak Ave, Peoria, IL 61637
Phone: (309) 655-3863
Fax: (309) 655-4161
Percentage of IMGs in the program: 40%
Minimum USMLE Step 1 Score Requirement: No limits set
Minimum USMLE Step 2 Score Requirement: No limits set

Attempts on any step: Must pass on first attempt
CS required at time of application: Yes
USCE Requirement: None
Cut-Off time since graduation: 5 years unless clinically active
Program offers couple match: Yes
Visas Sponsored or accepted: J1 visa and H1b visa

Loyola University Combined Med-Peds Residency Program

Specialty: Combined Internal Medicine/Pediatrics
Program name: Loyola University Program
Program code: 700-16-14-014
NRMP Code: 1170700C0
Program type: University-based
State: Illinois
Address: Loyola University Medical Center, Building 105 Room 3327,
          2160 S First Ave, Maywood, IL 60153
Phone: (708) 216-3145
Fax: (708) 327-9123
Percentage of IMGs in the program: 0%
Minimum USMLE Step 1 Score Requirement: 210
Minimum USMLE Step 2 Score Requirement: 210

Attempts on any step: Must pass on first attempt
CS required at time of application: No
USCE Requirement: None
Cut-Off time since graduation: 5 years
Program offers couple match: Yes
Visas Sponsored or accepted: J1 visa

Rush University Medical Center Combined Med-Peds Residency Program

Specialty: Combined Internal Medicine/Pediatrics
Program name: Rush University Medical Center Program
Program code: 700-16-32-103
NRMP Code: 1147700C0
Program type: University-based
State: Illinois
Address: Rush Lifetime Med Associates, Suite 215,
        1645 W Jackson Blvd, Chicago, IL 60612
Phone: (312) 942-3254
Fax: (312) 942-3551
Percentage of IMGs in the program: 0%
Minimum USMLE Step 1 Score Requirement: No limits set

Minimum USMLE Step 2 Score Requirement:
No limits set
Attempts on any step: No limits set
CS required at time of application: No
USCE Requirement: Yes
Cut-Off time since graduation: No limits et
Program offers couple match: Yes
Visas Sponsored or accepted: No visa

University of Illinois College of Medicine at Chicago Combined Med-Peds Residency Program

Specialty: Combined Internal
Medicine/Pediatrics
Program name: University of Illinois College of
Medicine at Chicago Program
Program code: 700-16-14-013
NRMP Code: 1150700C0
Program type: University-based
State: Illinois
Address: University of Illinois Hospital, Room
1405,
        840 S Wood St, Chicago, IL 60612-
7323
Phone: (312) 413-3803
Fax: (312) 413-0243
Percentage of IMGs in the program: 0%
Minimum USMLE Step 1 Score Requirement:
213

Minimum USMLE Step 2 Score Requirement: 210
Attempts on any step: Must pass on first attempt
CS required at time of application: No
USCE Requirement: None
Cut-Off time since graduation: 5 years
Program offers couple match: Yes
Visas Sponsored or accepted: J1 visa

University of Chicago Combined Med-Peds Residency Program

Specialty: Combined Internal Medicine/Pediatrics
Program name: University of Chicago Program
Program code: 700-16-14-012
NRMP Code: 1160700C0
Program type: University-based
State: Illinois
Address: University of Chicago Medical Center, MC7082,
            5841 S Maryland Ave, Chicago, IL 60637-1470
Phone: (773) 702-0309
Fax: (773) 702-2230
Percentage of IMGs in the program: 0%
Minimum USMLE Step 1 Score Requirement: No limits set

Minimum USMLE Step 2 Score Requirement:
No limits set
Attempts on any step: Maximum 2 attempts on
each step allowed
CS required at time of application: No
USCE Requirement: Yes, 3 months.
Cut-Off time since graduation: No limits set
Program offers couple match: Yes
Visas Sponsored or accepted: J1 visa

Indiana

Indiana University School of Medicine Combined Internal Medicine/Pediatrics Residency Program

Specialty: Combined Internal
Medicine/Pediatrics
Program name: Indiana University School of
Medicine Program
Program code: 700-17-14-018
NRMP Code: 1187700C0
Program type: University-based
State: Indiana
Address: Riley Hospital for Children, Room 5867
705 Riley Hospital Dr, Indianapolis, IN
46202-5225

Phone: (317) 948-0003
Fax: (317) 944-1476
Percentage of IMGs in the program: 0%
Minimum USMLE Step 1 Score Requirement: 220
Minimum USMLE Step 2 Score Requirement: 220
Attempts on any step: Must pass on first attempt including CS exam
CS required at time of application: No
USCE Requirement: Yes
Cut-Off time since graduation: No limits set
Program offers couple match: Yes
Visas Sponsored or accepted: J1 visa

Kansas

University of Kansas (Wichita) Combined Med-Peds Residency Program

Specialty: Combined Internal Medicine/Pediatrics
Program name: University of Kansas (Wichita) Program
Program code: 700-19-32-124
NRMP Code: 3054700C0

Program type: Community-based university affiliated hospital
State: Kansas
Address: University of Kansas School of Medicine-Wichita, Internal Medicine/Pediatrics, 550 N Hillside, Wichita, KS 67214
Phone: (316) 962-2212
Fax: (316) 962-7231
Percentage of IMGs in the program: 35%
Minimum USMLE Step 1 Score Requirement: No limits set
Minimum USMLE Step 2 Score Requirement: No limits set
Attempts on any step: Maximum of 2 attempts allowed on each step including the CS exam.
CS required at time of application: Yes including ECFMG certificate.
USCE Requirement: None
Cut-Off time since graduation: 5 years
Program offers couple match: Yes
Visas Sponsored or accepted: J1 visa

Kentucky

University of Louisville Combined Med-Peds Residency Program

Specialty: Combined Internal Medicine/Pediatrics
Program name: University of Louisville Program
Program code: 700-20-32-020
NRMP Code: 1217700C0
Program type: Community-based university affiliated hospital
State: Kentucky
Address: University of Louisville Hospital, Med-Peds Program A3K00,
　　　　 550 S Jackson St, Louisville, KY 40202
Phone: (502) 852-4277
Fax: (502) 852-8980
Percentage of IMGs in the program: 0%
Minimum USMLE Step 1 Score Requirement: No limits set
Minimum USMLE Step 2 Score Requirement: No limits set
Attempts on any step: No limits set
CS required at time of application: No
USCE Requirement: Yes
Cut-Off time since graduation: 3 years
Program offers couple match: Yes
Visas Sponsored or accepted: J1 visa

University of Kentucky College of Medicine Combined Med-Peds Residency Program

Specialty: Combined Internal Medicine/Pediatrics
Program name: University of Kentucky College of Medicine Program
Program code: 700-20-14-019
NRMP Code: 1848700C0
Program type: University-based
State: Kentucky
Address: University of Kentucky-Chandler Medical Center, 304B CTW Building,
        900 S Limestone St, Lexington, KY 40536-0200
Phone: (859) 323-6561
Fax: (859) 323-1197
Percentage of IMGs in the program: 0%
Minimum USMLE Step 1 Score Requirement: No limits set
Minimum USMLE Step 2 Score Requirement: No limits set
Attempts on any step: Must pass on first attempt on any step
CS required at time of application: No
USCE Requirement: Yes
Cut-Off time since graduation: 5 years
Program offers couple match: Yes

Visas Sponsored or accepted: J1 visa

Louisiana

Louisiana State University (Shreveport) Combined Med-Peds Residency Program

Specialty: Combined Internal Medicine/Pediatrics
Program name: Louisiana State University (Shreveport) Program
Program code: 700-21-32-101
NRMP Code: 1232700C0
Program type: University-based
State: Louisiana
Address: LSU Health Science Center Shreveport, Department of Medicine,
        1501 Kings Hwy, Shreveport, LA 71130
Phone: (318) 675-5915
Fax: (318) 675-5988
Percentage of IMGs in the program: 60%
Minimum USMLE Step 1 Score Requirement: No limits set
Minimum USMLE Step 2 Score Requirement: No limits set

Attempts on any step: Must pass on first attempt including CS exam
CS required at time of application: Yes
USCE Requirement: Yes
Cut-Off time since graduation: 5 years
Program offers couple match: Yes
Visas Sponsored or accepted: J1 visa

Louisiana State University Combined Med-Peds Residency Program

Specialty: Combined Internal Medicine/Pediatrics
Program name: Louisiana State University Program
Program code: 700-21-14-022
Program type: University-based
State: Louisiana
Address: LSU Health Science Center New Orleans, Box T4M-2 4th Floor Room 441A,
        1542 Tulane Ave, New Orleans, LA 70112
Phone: (504) 568-3792
Fax: (504) 568-2127
Percentage of IMGs in the program: 85%
Minimum USMLE Step 1 Score Requirement: 210
Minimum USMLE Step 2 Score Requirement: 210

Attempts on any step: Must pass on first attempt
CS required at time of application: Yes including ECFMG Certificate
USCE Requirement: Yes
Cut-Off time since graduation: 2 years
Program offers couple match: Yes
Visas Sponsored or accepted: J1 visa

Tulane University Combined Med-Peds Residency Program

Specialty: Combined Internal Medicine/Pediatrics
Program name: Tulane University Program
Program code: 700-21-32-023
NRMP Code: 3073700C0
Program type: University-based
State: Louisiana
Address: Tulane University Health Sciences Center, Box SL 37,
    1430 Tulane Ave, New Orleans, LA 70112
Phone: (504) 988-6689
Fax: (504) 988-6808
Percentage of IMGs in the program: 0%
Minimum USMLE Step 1 Score Requirement: No limits set

Minimum USMLE Step 2 Score Requirement: No limits set
Attempts on any step: No limits set
CS required at time of application: Yes as well as ECFMG certificate
USCE Requirement: Yes
Cut-Off time since graduation: 5 years
Program offers couple match: Yes
Visas Sponsored or accepted: J1 visa

Maine

Maine Medical Center Combined Med-Peds Residency Program

Specialty: Internal Medicine/Pediatrics
Program name: Maine Medical Center Program
Program code: 700-22-32-128
NRMP Code: 1236700C0
Program type: Community-based university affiliated hospital
State: Maine
Address: Maine Medical Center, Department of Pediatrics,
      22 Bramhall St, Portland, ME 04102
Phone: (207) 662-2405
Percentage of IMGs in the program: 0%
Minimum USMLE Step 1 Score Requirement: 210

Minimum USMLE Step 2 Score Requirement: 210
Attempts on any step: Must pass on first attempt
CS required at time of application: No
USCE Requirement: Yes 1-2 months
Cut-Off time since graduation: No limits set
Program offers couple match: Yes
Visas Sponsored or accepted: J1 visa

Maryland

Johns Hopkins University School of Medicine Combined Med-Peds Residency Program

Specialty: Combined Internal Medicine/Pediatrics
Program name: Johns Hopkins University School of Medicine Program
Program code: 700-23-14-143
Program type: University-based
State: Maryland
Address: Johns Hopkins Hospital, Suite 7143, 601 N Caroline St, Baltimore, MD 21287-0941
Phone: (410) 955-3613
Fax: (410) 614-1195
Percentage of IMGs in the program: 0%

Minimum USMLE Step 1 Score Requirement:
No limits set
Minimum USMLE Step 2 Score Requirement:
No limits set
Attempts on any step: Must pass on first attempt
CS required at time of application: No
USCE Requirement: None
Cut-Off time since graduation: 3 years
Program offers couple match: Yes
Visas Sponsored or accepted: H1b visa

University of Maryland Combined Med-Peds Residency Program

Specialty: Combined Internal Medicine/Pediatrics
Program name: University of Maryland Program
Program code: 700-23-32-095
NRMP Code: 1252700C0
Program type: University-based
State: Maryland
Address: University of Maryland Medical Center, Room N3E09,
            22 S Greene St, Baltimore, MD 21201-1595
Phone: (410) 328-2388
Percentage of IMGs in the program: 0%
Minimum USMLE Step 1 Score Requirement: 220

Minimum USMLE Step 2 Score Requirement: 220
Attempts on any step: No limits set
CS required at time of application: Yes including ECFMG certificate
USCE Requirement: Yes, 4 months
Cut-Off time since graduation: No limits set
Program offers couple match: Yes
Visas Sponsored or accepted: J1 visa

Massachusetts

University of Massachusetts Combined Med-Peds Residency Program

Specialty: Combined Internal Medicine/Pediatrics
Program name: University of Massachusetts Program
Program code: 700-24-32-111
NRMP Code: 3050700C0
Program type: University-based
State: Massachusetts
Address: University of Massachusetts Medical School, Internal Med/Peds Program,
        55 Lake Ave N, Worcester, MA 01655
Phone: (508) 856-7595

Fax: (774) 442-3779
Percentage of IMGs in the program: 0%
Minimum USMLE Step 1 Score Requirement:
No limits set
Minimum USMLE Step 2 Score Requirement:
No limits set
Attempts on any step: No limits set
CS required at time of application: No
USCE Requirement: Yes
Cut-Off time since graduation: No limits set
Program offers couple match: Yes
Visas Sponsored or accepted: J1 visa

Baystate Medical Center/Tufts University School of Medicine Combined Med-Peds Residency Program

Specialty: Combined Internal Medicine/Pediatrics
Program name: Baystate Medical Center/Tufts University School of Medicine Program
Program code: 700-24-32-024
NRMP Code: 1286700C0
Program type: Community-based university affiliated hospital
State: Massachusetts
Address: Baystate Medical Center, Room S2575, 759 Chestnut St, Springfield, MA 01199

Phone: (413) 794-3998
Fax: (413) 794-4588
Percentage of IMGs in the program: 0%
Minimum USMLE Step 1 Score Requirement: No limits set
Minimum USMLE Step 2 Score Requirement: No limits set
Attempts on any step: No limits set
CS required at time of application: No
USCE Requirement: Yes
Cut-Off time since graduation: 3 years
Program offers couple match: Yes
Visas Sponsored or accepted: J1 visa and H1b visa

Massachusetts General Hospital/Harvard Medical School Combined Med-Peds Residency Program

Specialty: Combined Internal Medicine/Pediatrics
Program name: Massachusetts General Hospital/Harvard Medical School Program
Program code: 700-24-14-097
NRMP Code: 1261700C2
Program type: University-based
State: Massachusetts
Address: Massachusetts General Hospital for Children, 5th Floor,

175 Cambridge St, Boston, MA 02114
Phone: (617) 726-7782
Fax: (617) 724-9068
Percentage of IMGs in the program: 0%
Minimum USMLE Step 1 Score Requirement:
No limits set
Minimum USMLE Step 2 Score Requirement:
No limits set
Attempts on any step: No limits set
CS required at time of application: No
USCE Requirement: None
Cut-Off time since graduation: No limits set
Program offers couple match: Yes
Visas Sponsored or accepted: J1 visa and H1b
visa

Brigham and Women Hospital/Children Hospital/Harvard Medical School Combined Med-Peds Residency Program

Specialty: Combined Internal
Medicine/Pediatrics
Program name: Brigham and Women's
Hospital/Children's Hospital/Harvard Medical
School
Program
Program code: 700-24-14-084

NRMP Code: 1265700C0
Program type: University-based
State: Massachusetts
Address: Brigham and Women's Hospital,
Internal Medicine/Pediatrics Program,
       75 Francis St, Boston, MA 02115
Phone: (617) 525-7278
Fax: (617) 264-6346
Percentage of IMGs in the program: 0%
Minimum USMLE Step 1 Score Requirement:
No limits set
Minimum USMLE Step 2 Score Requirement:
No limits set
Attempts on any step: Must pass on first
attempt
CS required at time of application: No
USCE Requirement: Yes, 1 month
Cut-Off time since graduation: No limits set
Program offers couple match: Yes
Visas Sponsored or accepted: J1 and H1b visa

Michigan

William Beaumont Hospital Combined Med-Peds Residency Program

Specialty: Combined Internal Medicine/Pediatrics
Program name: William Beaumont Hospital Program
Program code: 700-25-32-033
NRMP Code: 1978700C0
Program type: Community-based university affiliated hospital
State: Michigan
Address: William Beaumont Hospital, Med/Peds Program,
3601 W 13 Mile Rd, Royal Oak, MI 48073-6769
Phone: (248) 551-6489
Fax: (248) 551-8880
Percentage of IMGs in the program: 50%
Minimum USMLE Step 1 Score Requirement: 210
Minimum USMLE Step 2 Score Requirement: 210
Attempts on any step: No limits set
CS required at time of application: No
USCE Requirement: None
Cut-Off time since graduation: No limits set
Program offers couple match: Yes
Visas Sponsored or accepted: J1 visa and H1b visa

Western Michigan University School of Medicine Combined Med-Peds Residency Program

Specialty: Combined Internal Medicine/Pediatrics
Program name: Western Michigan University School of Medicine Program
Program code: 700-25-14-089
NRMP Code: 1314700C0
Program type: Community-based university affiliated hospital
State: Michigan
Address: Western Michigan University School of Medicine, Med/Peds Program
            1000 Oakland Dr, Kalamazoo, MI 49008
Phone: (269) 337-6353
Fax: (269) 337-4262
Percentage of IMGs in the program: 20%
Minimum USMLE Step 1 Score Requirement: 225
Minimum USMLE Step 2 Score Requirement: 225
Attempts on any step: Must pass on first attempt
CS required at time of application: No
USCE Requirement: None
Cut-Off time since graduation: 5 years unless clinically active like in residency or clinical practice

Program offers couple match: Yes
Visas Sponsored or accepted: J1 visa and H1b visa

Grand Rapids Medical Education Partners/Michigan State University Combined Med-Peds Residency Program

Specialty: Combined Internal Medicine/Pediatrics
Program name: Grand Rapids Medical Education Partners/Michigan State University Program
Program code: 700-25-14-098
NRMP Code: 2077700C0
Program type: Community-based university affiliated hospital
State: Michigan
Address: Grand Rapids Medical Education Partners, Suite 2200,
         25 Michigan Ave NE, Grand Rapids, MI 49503
Phone: (616) 391-3776
Fax: (616) 391-3130
Percentage of IMGs in the program: 0%
Minimum USMLE Step 1 Score Requirement: 220
Minimum USMLE Step 2 Score Requirement: 220

Attempts on any step: Must pass on first attempt including the CS exam
CS required at time of application: No
USCE Requirement: Yes
Cut-Off time since graduation: 3 years
Program offers couple match: Yes
Visas Sponsored or accepted: J1 visa

Hurley Medical Center/Michigan State University Combined Med-Peds Residency Program

Specialty: Combined Internal Medicine/Pediatrics
Program name: Hurley Medical Center/Michigan State University Program
Program code: 700-25-32-030
NRMP Code: 1307700C0
Program type: Community-based university affiliated hospital
State: Michigan
Address: Hurley Medical Center, Combined Med-Peds Education 3AW,
            One Hurley Plaza, Flint, MI 48503
Phone: (810) 262-9283
Fax: (810) 262-9736
Percentage of IMGs in the program: 10%
Minimum USMLE Step 1 Score Requirement: 206

Minimum USMLE Step 2 Score Requirement: 206
Attempts on any step: No limits set
CS required at time of application: Yes as well as ECFMG certificate
USCE Requirement: None
Cut-Off time since graduation: 5 years unless clinically active as residency or clinical practice.
Program offers couple match: Yes
Visas Sponsored or accepted: J1 visa and H1b visa

Detroit Medical Center/Wayne State University Combined Med-Peds Residency Program

Specialty: Combined Internal Medicine/Pediatrics
Program name: Detroit Medical Center/Wayne State University Program
Program code: 700-25-14-029
NRMP Code: 1295700C0
Program type: University-based
State: Michigan
Address: Wayne State University/Detroit Medical Center, UHC 2E,
          4201 St Antoine Blvd, Detroit, MI 48201
Phone: (313) 577-4342

Fax: (313) 745-4052
Percentage of IMGs in the program: 0%
Minimum USMLE Step 1 Score Requirement:
No limits set
Minimum USMLE Step 2 Score Requirement:
No limits set
Attempts on any step: Must pass on first
attempt
CS required at time of application: Yes
USCE Requirement: None
Cut-Off time since graduation: 3 years
Program offers couple match: Yes
Visas Sponsored or accepted: J1 visa

University of Michigan Combined Med-Peds Residency Program

Specialty: Combined Internal
Medicine/Pediatrics
Program name: University of Michigan Program
Program code: 700-25-14-025
NRMP Code: 1293700C0
Program type: University-based
State: Michigan
Address: University of Michigan Hospitals and
Health Centers, 3116 Taubman Ctr SPC 5368,
            1500 E Medical Center Drive, Ann
Arbor, MI 48109-5368
Phone: (734) 936-4385
Fax: (734) 936-3654

Percentage of IMGs in the program: 0%
Minimum USMLE Step 1 Score Requirement:
No limits set
Minimum USMLE Step 2 Score Requirement:
No limits set
Attempts on any step: No limits set
CS required at time of application: No
USCE Requirement: Yes
Cut-Off time since graduation: No limits set
Program offers couple match: Yes
Visas Sponsored or accepted: J1 visa

Minnesota

University of Minnesota Combined Med/Peds Residency Program

Specialty: Combined Internal
Medicine/Pediatrics
Program name: University of Minnesota
Program
Program code: 700-26-14-034
NRMP Code: 1334700C0
Program type: University-based
State: Minnesota

Address: University of Minnesota Medical School, MMC 913,

420 Delaware St SE, Minneapolis, MN 55455-0392

Phone: (612) 624-0990

Fax: (612) 625-3238

Percentage of IMGs in the program: 0%

Minimum USMLE Step 1 Score Requirement: 190

Minimum USMLE Step 2 Score Requirement: 205

Attempts on any step: Must pass on first attempt

CS required at time of application: Yes as well as ECFMG certificate

USCE Requirement: Yes, preferably 1 months onsite or affiliated clinic.

Cut-Off time since graduation: No limits set

Program offers couple match: Yes

Visas Sponsored or accepted: J1 visa

Mississippi

University of Mississippi Medical Center Combined Med-Peds Residency Program

Specialty: Combined Internal Medicine/Pediatrics
Program name: University of Mississippi Medical Center Program
Program code: 700-27-14-035
NRMP Code: 1957700C0
Program type: University-based
State: Mississippi
Address: University of Mississippi Medical Center, Department of Medicine,
          2500 N State St, Jackson, MS 39216-4505
Phone: (601) 984-5532
Fax: (601) 984-6665
Percentage of IMGs in the program: 0%
Minimum USMLE Step 1 Score Requirement: No limits set
Minimum USMLE Step 2 Score Requirement: No limits set
Attempts on any step: Maximum of two attempts on each step
CS required at time of application: No
USCE Requirement: None
Cut-Off time since graduation: No limits set
Program offers couple match: Yes
Visas Sponsored or accepted: J1 visa

Missouri

St. Louis University School of Medicine Combined Med/Peds Residency Program

Specialty: Combined Internal Medicine/Pediatrics
Program name: St Louis University School of Medicine Program
Program code: 700-28-14-037
Program type: University-based
State: Missouri
Address: St Louis University School of Medicine, Department of Internal Medicine,
          1402 S Grand Blvd, St Louis, MO 63104
Phone: (314) 577-8762
Fax: (314) 268-5108
Percentage of IMGs in the program: 40%
Minimum USMLE Step 1 Score Requirement: 212
Minimum USMLE Step 2 Score Requirement: 212
Attempts on any step: Must pass on first attempt
CS required at time of application: No
USCE Requirement: Yes
Cut-Off time since graduation: 5 years
Program offers couple match: Yes

Visas Sponsored or accepted: J1 visa and H1b visa

University of Missouri at Kansas City Combined Med-Peds Residency Program

Specialty: Combined Internal Medicine/Pediatrics
Program name: University of Missouri at Kansas City Program
Program code: 700-28-32-036
NRMP Code: 1343700C0
Program type: University-based
State: Missouri
Address: UMKC School of Med, Medicine/Pediatrics Program,
        2411 Holmes St, Kansas City, MO 64108
Phone: (816) 404-0525
Fax: (816) 404-0959
Percentage of IMGs in the program: 0%
Minimum USMLE Step 1 Score Requirement: No limits set
Minimum USMLE Step 2 Score Requirement: No limits set
Attempts on any step: Must pass on first attempt
CS required at time of application: No
USCE Requirement: Yes

Cut-Off time since graduation: 2 years
Program offers couple match: Yes
Visas Sponsored or accepted: No visa

University of Missouri-Columbia Combined Med-Peds Residency Program

Specialty: Combined Internal Medicine/Pediatrics
Program name: University of Missouri-Columbia Program
Program code: 700-28-32-126
NRMP Code: 1994700C0
Program type: University-based
State: Missouri
Address: University of Missouri Hospitals and Clinics, Department of Child Health DCO5800, One Hospital Dr, Columbia, MO 65212
Phone:(573) 882-4438
Fax: (573) 884-9992
Percentage of IMGs in the program: 0%
Minimum USMLE Step 1 Score Requirement: 210
Minimum USMLE Step 2 Score Requirement: 210
Attempts on any step: Must pass on first attempt including CS exam
CS required at time of application: Yes including ECFMG certificate

USCE Requirement: None
Cut-Off time since graduation: 3 years
Program offers couple match: Yes
Visas Sponsored or accepted: J1 visa

Nebraska

University of Nebraska Medical Center College of Medicine Combined Med-Peds Residency Program

Specialty: Combined Internal Medicine/Pediatrics
Program name: University of Nebraska Medical Center College of Medicine Program
Program code: 700-30-14-136
NRMP Code: 1376700C0
Program type: University-based
State: Nebraska
Address: University of Nebraska Medical Center, Department of Internal Medicine Education,

982055 Nebraska Med Center,
Omaha, NE 68198-2055
Phone: (402) 559-7792
Fax: (402) 559-9385
Percentage of IMGs in the program: 15%
Minimum USMLE Step 1 Score Requirement:
205
Minimum USMLE Step 2 Score Requirement:
205
Attempts on any step: Must pass on first
attempt
CS required at time of application: No
USCE Requirement: None
Cut-Off time since graduation: No limits set
Program offers couple match: Yes
Visas Sponsored or accepted: J1 visa and H1b
visa

New Jersey

Newark Beth Israel Medical Center Combined Med-Peds Residency Program

Specialty: Combined Internal
Medicine/Pediatrics
Program name: Newark Beth Israel Medical
Center Program

Program code: 700-33-32-041
State: New Jersey
Address: Newark Beth Israel Medical Center, Medicine-Pediatrics,
          201 Lyons Ave, Newark, NJ 07112
Phone: (973) 926-4949
Fax: (973) 923-2441
Percentage of IMGs in the program: 40%
Minimum USMLE Step 1 Score Requirement: 210
Minimum USMLE Step 2 Score Requirement: 210
Attempts on any step: No limits set
CS required at time of application: No
USCE Requirement: None
Cut-Off time since graduation: 2 years
Program offers couple match: Yes
Visas Sponsored or accepted: No visa

UMDNJ-New Jersey Medical School Combined Med-Peds Residency Program

Specialty: Combined Internal Medicine/Pediatrics
Program name: Rutgers New Jersey Medical School Program
Program code: 700-33-32-040
NRMP Code: 1398700C0

Program type: University-based
State: New Jersey
Address: Rutgers New Jersey Medical School, UH I-247,
    150 Bergen St, Newark, NJ 07103
Phone: (973) 972-6056
Fax: (973) 972-3129
Percentage of IMGs in the program: 30%
Minimum USMLE Step 1 Score Requirement: No limits set
Minimum USMLE Step 2 Score Requirement: No limits set
Attempts on any step: No limits set
CS required at time of application: No
USCE Requirement: None
Cut-Off time since graduation: No limits set
Program offers couple match: Yes
Visas Sponsored or accepted: J1 visa

New York

Mount Sinai School of Medicine Combined Med-Peds Residency Program

Specialty: Combined Internal Medicine/Pediatrics

Program name: Icahn School of Medicine at Mount Sinai Program
Program code: 700-35-32-105
State: New York
Address: Mount Sinai Medical Center, Box 1512,
          One Gustave L Levy Pl, New York, NY 10029
Phone: (212) 241-6934
Fax: (212) 241-4309
Percentage of IMGs in the program: 0%
Minimum USMLE Step 1 Score Requirement: No limits set
Minimum USMLE Step 2 Score Requirement: No limits set
Attempts on any step: No limits set
CS required at time of application: No
USCE Requirement: None
Cut-Off time since graduation: No limits set
Program offers couple match: Yes
Visas Sponsored or accepted: J1 visa and H1b visa

SUNY at Stony Brook Combined Med-Peds Residency Program

Specialty: Combined Internal Medicine/Pediatrics
Program name: SUNY at Stony Brook Program
Program code: 700-35-32-093

NRMP Code: 2919700C0
Program type: University-based
State: New York
Address: SUNY Stony Brook University, Internal Medicine/Pediatrics Program,

HSC T-11 040, Stony Brook, NY 11794-8111
Phone: (631) 444-2020
Percentage of IMGs in the program: 20%
Minimum USMLE Step 1 Score Requirement: No limits set
Minimum USMLE Step 2 Score Requirement: No limits set
Attempts on any step: Must pass on first attempt including CS exam
CS required at time of application: Yes
USCE Requirement: None
Cut-Off time since graduation: 10 years
Program offers couple match: Yes
Visas Sponsored or accepted: J1 visa

University of Rochester Combined Med-Peds Residency Program

Specialty: Combined Internal Medicine/Pediatrics
Program name: University of Rochester Program
Program code: 700-35-32-054
NRMP Code: 1511700C0

Program type: University-based
State: New York
Address: University of Rochester Medical Center, Box 777R,
          601 Elmwood Ave, Rochester, NY 14642
Phone: (585) 273-1044
Fax: (585) 442-6580
Percentage of IMGs in the program: 0%
Minimum USMLE Step 1 Score Requirement: 220
Minimum USMLE Step 2 Score Requirement: 220
Attempts on any step: No limits set
CS required at time of application: No
USCE Requirement: Yes, 2 months
Cut-Off time since graduation: 10 years
Program offers couple match: No
Visas Sponsored or accepted: J1 visa

Albany Medical Center Combined Med-Peds Residency Program

Specialty: Combined Internal Medicine/Pediatrics
Program name: Albany Medical Center Program
Program code: 700-35-14-044
NRMP Code: 1414700C0
Program type: University-based
State: New York

Address: Albany Medical Center, Internal Medicine/Pediatrics Program,
        724 Watervliet-Shaker Rd, Latham, NY 12110
Phone: (518) 262-7585
Fax: (518) 262-7505
Percentage of IMGs in the program: 20%
Minimum USMLE Step 1 Score Requirement: No limits set
Minimum USMLE Step 2 Score Requirement: No limits set
Attempts on any step: Must pass on first attempt
CS required at time of application: No
USCE Requirement: Yes
Cut-Off time since graduation: 5 years unless clinically active as in residency or practice.
Program offers couple match: Yes
Visas Sponsored or accepted: J1 visa

University at Buffalo Combined Med-Peds Residency Program

Specialty: Combined Internal Medicine/Pediatrics
Program name: University at Buffalo Program
Program code: 700-35-32-049
NRMP Code: 3099700C0
Program type: Community-based university affiliated hospital

State: New York
Address: Women and Children's Hospital
Buffalo, Division of Internal Medicine-Pediatrics,
300 Linwood Ave, Buffalo, NY 14209
Phone: (716) 961-9412
Fax: (716) 961-9403
Percentage of IMGs in the program: 40%
Minimum USMLE Step 1 Score Requirement:
205
Minimum USMLE Step 2 Score Requirement:
205
Attempts on any step: Must pass on first
attempt
CS required at time of application: No
USCE Requirement: Yes
Cut-Off time since graduation: 2 years
Program offers couple match: Yes
Visas Sponsored or accepted: J1 visa

North Carolina

Vidant Medical Center/East Carolina University Combined Med-Peds Residency Program

Specialty: Combined Internal
Medicine/Pediatrics

Program name: Vidant Medical Center/East Carolina University Program
Program code: 700-36-32-057
NRMP Code: 3057700C0
Program type: University-based
State: North Carolina
Address: Brody School of Medicine ECU, PCMH-MA 307,

        600 Moye Blvd, Greenville, NC 27834
Phone: (252) 744-3961
Fax: (252) 744-4688
Percentage of IMGs in the program: 15%
Minimum USMLE Step 1 Score Requirement: No limits set
Minimum USMLE Step 2 Score Requirement: No limits set
Attempts on any step: No limits set
CS required at time of application: No
USCE Requirement: None
Cut-Off time since graduation: 3 years
Program offers couple match: Yes
Visas Sponsored or accepted: J1 visa

Duke University Hospital Combined Med-Peds Residency Program

Specialty: Combined Internal Medicine/Pediatrics
Program name: Duke University Hospital Program

Program code: 700-36-14-056
NRMP Code:
Program type:
State: North Carolina
Address: Duke University Medical Center,
Department of Medicine-Pediatrics,
         Box 3127, Durham, NC 27710
Phone: (919) 681-3009
Fax: (919) 681-5825
Percentage of IMGs in the program: 5%
Minimum USMLE Step 1 Score Requirement:
No limits set
Minimum USMLE Step 2 Score Requirement:
No limits set
Attempts on any step: No limits set
CS required at time of application:
Yes including ECFMG certificate
USCE Requirement: None
Cut-Off time since graduation: No limits set
Program offers couple match: Yes
Visas Sponsored or accepted: J1 visa

University of North Carolina Hospitals Combined Med-Peds Residency Program

Specialty: Combined Internal
Medicine/Pediatrics
Program name: University of North Carolina
Hospitals Program

Program code: 700-36-32-055
NRMP Code: 1900700C0
Program type: University-based
State: North Carolina
Address: University of North Carolina Hospitals, 230 MacNider Hall,
CB#7593, Chapel Hill, NC 27599-7593
Phone: (919) 966-6770
Fax: (919) 966-8419
Percentage of IMGs in the program: 0%
Minimum USMLE Step 1 Score Requirement: No limits set
Minimum USMLE Step 2 Score Requirement: No limits set
Attempts on any step: Must pass on first attempt including CS exam
CS required at time of application: Yes as well as ECFMG certificate
USCE Requirement: Yes
Cut-Off time since graduation: 2 years
Program offers couple match: Yes
Visas Sponsored or accepted: J1 visa

Ohio

Ohio State University Hospital Combined Med-Peds Residency Program

Specialty: Combined Internal Medicine/Pediatrics
Program name: Ohio State University Hospital Program
Program code: 700-38-14-063
NRMP Code: 1566700C0
Program type: University-based
State: Ohio
Address: Nationwide Children's Hospital, Rm ED-650A,
            700 Children's Dr, Columbus, OH 43205
Phone: (614) 722-0417
Fax: (614) 722-6132
Percentage of IMGs in the program: 0% (occasionally 1 resident)
Minimum USMLE Step 1 Score Requirement: No limits set
Minimum USMLE Step 2 Score Requirement: No limits set
Attempts on any step: No limits set
CS required at time of application: Yes
USCE Requirement: Yes
Cut-Off time since graduation: 5 years
Program offers couple match: Yes
Visas Sponsored or accepted: J1 visa and H1b visa

Case Western Reserve University/University Hospitals Case Medical Center Combined Med-Peds Residency Program

Specialty: Combined Internal Medicine/Pediatrics
Program name: Case Western Reserve University/University Hospitals Case Medical Center Program
Program code: 700-38-32-121
NRMP Code: 1552700C0
Program type: University-based
State: Ohio
Address: University Hospitals Case Medical Center, Lakeside 1507,
        11100 Euclid Ave, Cleveland, OH 44106-6055
Phone: (216) 844-8431
Fax: (216) 844-7497
Percentage of IMGs in the program: 65%
Minimum USMLE Step 1 Score Requirement: No limits set
Minimum USMLE Step 2 Score Requirement: No limits set
Attempts on any step: No limits set
CS required at time of application: No
USCE Requirement: None
Cut-Off time since graduation: 3 years

Program offers couple match: Yes
Visas Sponsored or accepted: J1 visa

Case Western Reserve University (MetroHealth) Combined Med-Peds Residency Program

Specialty: Combined Internal Medicine/Pediatrics
Program name: Case Western Reserve University (MetroHealth) Program
Program code: 700-38-32-061
NRMP Code: 1553700C0
Program type: University-based
State: Ohio
Address: MetroHealth Medical Center, Internal Medicine-Pediatrics H574,
          2500 MetroHealth Dr, Cleveland, OH 44109-1998
Phone: (216) 778-2882
Fax: (216) 778-1384
Percentage of IMGs in the program: 35%
Minimum USMLE Step 1 Score Requirement: 210
Minimum USMLE Step 2 Score Requirement: 210
Attempts on any step: Must pass on first attempt including CS exam
CS required at time of application: No
USCE Requirement: None

Cut-Off time since graduation: 5 years
Program offers couple match: Yes
Visas Sponsored or accepted: J1 visa and H1b visa

University Hospital/University of Cincinnati College of Medicine Combined Med-Peds Residency Program

Specialty: Combined Internal Medicine/Pediatrics
Program name: University of Cincinnati Medical Center/College of Medicine Program
Program code: 700-38-14-082
NRMP Code: 1548700C0
Program type: University-based
State: Ohio
Address: University Hospital University of Cincinnati, Department of Internal Medicine,
        PO Box 670557, Cincinnati, OH 45267-0557
Phone: (513) 584-0397
Fax: (513) 584-0369
Percentage of IMGs in the program: 0%
Minimum USMLE Step 1 Score Requirement: No limits set
Minimum USMLE Step 2 Score Requirement: No limits set
Attempts on any step: No limits set

CS required at time of application: No
USCE Requirement: None
Cut-Off time since graduation: No limits set
Program offers couple match: Yes
Visas Sponsored or accepted: J1 visa

Oklahoma

University of Oklahoma College of Medicine-Tulsa Combined Med-Peds Residency Program

Specialty: Combined Internal Medicine/Pediatrics
Program name: University of Oklahoma College of Medicine-Tulsa Program
Program code: 700-39-32-067
State: Oklahoma
Address: University of Oklahoma Coll of Med-Tulsa, Sect of Med/Pediatrics #3G06,
          4502 E 41st St, Tulsa, OK 74135-2512
Phone: (918) 660-3395
Fax: (918) 660-3444
Percentage of IMGs in the program: 25%
Minimum USMLE Step 1 Score Requirement: 205
Minimum USMLE Step 2 Score Requirement: 205

Attempts on any step: No limits set
CS required at time of application: No
USCE Requirement: None
Cut-Off time since graduation: No limits set
Program offers couple match: Yes
Visas Sponsored or accepted: J1 visa and H1b visa

University of Oklahoma Health Sciences Center Combined Med-Peds Residency Program

Specialty: Combined Internal Medicine/Pediatrics
Program name: University of Oklahoma Health Sciences Center Program
Program code: 700-39-32-090
NRMP Code: 1588700C0
Program type: University-based
State: Oklahoma
Address: Children's Hospital Oklahoma City, A2 14000,
         1200 Children's Ave, Oklahoma City, OK 73104
Phone: (405) 271-4417
Fax: (405) 271-2920
Percentage of IMGs in the program: 60%
Minimum USMLE Step 1 Score Requirement: No limits set

Minimum USMLE Step 2 Score Requirement:
No limits set
Attempts on any step: No limits set
CS required at time of application: Yes
including ECFMG certificate
USCE Requirement: None
Cut-Off time since graduation: 3 years
Program offers couple match: Yes
Visas Sponsored or accepted: J1 visa

Pennsylvania

UPMC Medical Education Combined Med-Peds Residency Program

Specialty: Combined Internal
Medicine/Pediatrics
Program name: UPMC Medical Education
Program
Program code: 700-41-14-128
NRMP Code: 1652700C0
Program type: University-based
State: Pennsylvania
Address: University of Pittsburgh Medical
Center, N715 MUH,
          200 Lothrop St, Pittsburgh, PA 15213
Phone: (412) 683-7647
Fax: (412) 692-4944

Percentage of IMGs in the program: 0%
Minimum USMLE Step 1 Score Requirement:
No limits set
Minimum USMLE Step 2 Score Requirement:
No limits set
Attempts on any step: No limits set
CS required at time of application: Yes
including ECFMG certificate
USCE Requirement: None
Cut-Off time since graduation: No limits set
Program offers couple match: Yes
Visas Sponsored or accepted: J1 visa and H1b
visa

University of Pennsylvania Combined Med-Peds Residency Program

Specialty: Combined Internal
Medicine/Pediatrics
Program name: University of Pennsylvania
Program
Program code: 700-41-14-129
NRMP Code: 1628700C0
Program type: University-based
State: Pennsylvania
Address: University of Pennsylvania Health
System, 100 Centrex,
        3400 Spruce St, Philadelphia, PA
19104

Phone: (215) 662-2532
Fax: (215) 662-7919
Percentage of IMGs in the program: 0%
Minimum USMLE Step 1 Score Requirement: 210
Minimum USMLE Step 2 Score Requirement: 210
Attempts on any step: No limits set
CS required at time of application: No
USCE Requirement: Yes, 1 month
Cut-Off time since graduation: 4 years
Program offers couple match: Yes
Visas Sponsored or accepted: J1 visa and H1b visa

Penn State University/Milton S Hershey Medical Center Combined Med-Peds Residency Program

Specialty: Combined Internal Medicine/Pediatrics
Program name: Penn State Milton S Hershey Medical Center Program
Program code: 700-41-32-081
NRMP Code: 1617700C0
Program type: University-based
State: Pennsylvania
Address: Milton S Hershey Medical Center, PO Box 850 MC H085,

500 University Dr, Hershey, PA 17033-0850
Phone: (717) 531-8899
Fax: (717) 531-0856
Percentage of IMGs in the program: 10%
Minimum USMLE Step 1 Score Requirement: No limits set
Minimum USMLE Step 2 Score Requirement: No limits set
Attempts on any step: No limits set
CS required at time of application: No
USCE Requirement: None
Cut-Off time since graduation: 2 years
Program offers couple match: Yes
Visas Sponsored or accepted: J1 visa

Geisinger Health System Combined Med-Peds Residency Program

Specialty: Combined Internal Medicine/Pediatrics
Program name: Geisinger Health System Program
Program code: 700-41-14-068
NRMP Code: 1608700C0
Program type: Community-based university affiliated hospital
State: Pennsylvania
Address: Geisinger Medical Center, MC 01-38,

100 N Academy Ave, Danville, PA
17822-0138
Phone: (570) 271-6520
Fax: (570) 214-6354
Percentage of IMGs in the program: 30%
Minimum USMLE Step 1 Score Requirement:
No limits set
Minimum USMLE Step 2 Score Requirement:
No limits set
Attempts on any step: Must pass on first
attempt
CS required at time of application: No
USCE Requirement: None
Cut-Off time since graduation: No limits set
Program offers couple match: Yes
Visas Sponsored or accepted: J1 visa and H1b
visa

Rhode Island

Brown University Combined Med-Peds Residency Program

Specialty: Combined Internal
Medicine/Pediatrics
Program name: Brown University Program
Program code: 700-43-14-108

NRMP Code: 1677700C0
Program type: University-based
State: Rhode Island
Address: Rhode Island Hospital, Dept of
Med/Peds POB #224,
          593 Eddy St, Providence, RI 02903
Phone: (401) 444-4393
Fax: (401) 444-8804
Percentage of IMGs in the program: 0%
Minimum USMLE Step 1 Score Requirement:
210
Minimum USMLE Step 2 Score Requirement:
210
Attempts on any step: Must pass on first
attempt
CS required at time of application: No
USCE Requirement: None
Cut-Off time since graduation: No limits set
Program offers couple match: Yes
Visas Sponsored or accepted: J1 visa and H1b
visa

South Carolina

Greenville Hospital System/University of South Carolina Combined Med-Peds Residency Program

Specialty: Combined Internal Medicine/Pediatrics
Program name: Greenville Hospital System/University of South Carolina Program
Program code: 700-45-14-135
State: South Carolina
Address: Greenville Hospital System, Med-Peds Residency,
       701 Grove Rd, Greenville, SC 29605
Phone: (864) 455-7844
Fax: (864) 455-7848
Percentage of IMGs in the program: 0%
Minimum USMLE Step 1 Score Requirement: 210
Minimum USMLE Step 2 Score Requirement: 210
Attempts on any step: Must pass on first attempt
CS required at time of application: No
USCE Requirement: Yes
Cut-Off time since graduation: 3 years
Program offers couple match: Yes
Visas Sponsored or accepted: J1 visa

Medical University of South Carolina Combined Med-Peds Residency Program

Specialty: Combined Internal Medicine/Pediatrics
Program name: Medical University of South Carolina Program
Program code: 700-45-32-127
NRMP Code: 1680700C0
Program type: University-based
State: South Carolina
Address: Medical University of South Carolina, MSC 917 CH 688,
       165 Ashley Ave, Charleston, SC 29425
Phone: (843) 792-0435
Fax: (843) 792-9223
Percentage of IMGs in the program: 0%
Minimum USMLE Step 1 Score Requirement: 210
Minimum USMLE Step 2 Score Requirement: 210
Attempts on any step: No limits set
CS required at time of application: No
USCE Requirement: None
Cut-Off time since graduation: No limits set
Program offers couple match: Yes
Visas Sponsored or accepted: No visa

Tennessee

Vanderbilt University Combined Med-Peds Residency Program

Specialty: Combined Internal Medicine/Pediatrics
Program name: Vanderbilt University Program
Program code: 700-47-14-070
Program type: University-based
State: Tennessee
Address: Vanderbilt Univ Med Ctr
Ste 6000 Med Ctr East North Tower
1215 21st Ave S
Nashville, TN 37232-8300
Phone: (615) 936-8590
Fax: (615) 936-1269
Percentage of IMGs in the program: 0%
Minimum USMLE Step 1 Score Requirement: 220
Minimum USMLE Step 2 Score Requirement: 220
Attempts on any step: No limits set
CS required at time of application: Yes including ECFMG certificate
USCE Requirement: Yes
Cut-Off time since graduation: No limits set
Program offers couple match: Yes
Visas Sponsored or accepted: J1 visa

University of Tennessee Combined Med-Peds Residency Program

Specialty: Combined Internal Medicine/Pediatrics
Program name: University of Tennessee Program
Program code: 700-47-32-071
NRMP Code: 1844700C0
Program type: University-based
State: Tennessee
Address: University of Tennessee Medical Center, Room H316,
          956 Court Ave, Memphis, TN 38163
Phone: (901) 448-3714
Fax: (901) 448-7836
Percentage of IMGs in the program: 8%
Minimum USMLE Step 1 Score Requirement: 210
Minimum USMLE Step 2 Score Requirement: 210
Attempts on any step: Must pass on first attempt
CS required at time of application: No
USCE Requirement: Yes, 3 months
Cut-Off time since graduation: 5 years unless clinically active as in residency or practice
Program offers couple match: Yes
Visas Sponsored or accepted: J1 visa

Texas

University of Texas at Houston Combined Med-Peds Residency Program

Specialty: Combined Internal Medicine/Pediatrics
Program name: University of Texas at Houston Program
Program code: 700-48-14-075
NRMP Code: 2923700C0
Program type: University-based
State: Texas
Address: University of Texas Medical School Houston, Department of Internal Medicine Suite 1126,
            6431 Fannin St, Houston, TX 77030
Phone: (713) 500-6525
Fax: (713) 500-6530
Percentage of IMGs in the program: 0%
Minimum USMLE Step 1 Score Requirement: No limits set
Minimum USMLE Step 2 Score Requirement: No limits set
Attempts on any step: Must pass on first attempt including CS exam
CS required at time of application: No
USCE Requirement: Yes
Cut-Off time since graduation: 3 years

Program offers couple match: Yes
Visas Sponsored or accepted: J1 visa

Baylor College of Medicine Combined Med-Peds Residency Program

Specialty: Combined Internal Medicine/Pediatrics
Program name: Baylor College of Medicine Program
Program code: 700-48-14-074
NRMP Code: 1716700C0
Program type: University-based
State: Texas
Address: Baylor College of Medicine, Baylor Clinic Ste 1100-D,
        6620 Main St, Houston, TX 77030
Phone: (713) 798-0104
Fax: (713) 798-0223
Percentage of IMGs in the program: 0%
Minimum USMLE Step 1 Score Requirement: 220
Minimum USMLE Step 2 Score Requirement: 220
Attempts on any step: Must pass on first attempt
CS required at time of application: Yes including ECFMG certificate
USCE Requirement: None

Cut-Off time since graduation: 5 years
Program offers couple match: Yes
Visas Sponsored or accepted: No visa

Utah

University of Utah Combined Med-Peds Residency Program

Specialty: Combined Internal Medicine/Pediatrics
Program name: University of Utah Program
Program code: 700-49-14-091
NRMP Code: 1732700C0
Program type: University-based
State: Utah
Address: University of Utah Medical Center, Medicine/Pediatrics Program Rm 4C116,
          30 N 1900 E, Salt Lake City, UT 84132
Phone: (801) 585-5559
Fax: (801) 585-0418
Percentage of IMGs in the program: 0%
Minimum USMLE Step 1 Score Requirement: No limits set
Minimum USMLE Step 2 Score Requirement: No limits set
Attempts on any step: No limits set
CS required at time of application: No

USCE Requirement: Yes
Cut-Off time since graduation: 5 years
Program offers couple match: Yes
Visas Sponsored or accepted: J1 visa

Virginia

Virginia Commonwealth University Health System Combined Med-Peds Residency Program

Specialty: Combined Internal Medicine/Pediatrics
Program name: Virginia Commonwealth University Health System Program
Program code: 700-51-32-077
NRMP Code: 1743700C0
Program type: University-based
State: Virginia
Address: Virginia Commonwealth University Health System, Box 980163,
1101 E Marshall St, Richmond, VA 23298-0163
Phone: (804) 828-1808
Fax: (804) 827-0503
Percentage of IMGs in the program: 0%
Minimum USMLE Step 1 Score Requirement: No limits set

Minimum USMLE Step 2 Score Requirement:
No limits set
Attempts on any step: No limits set
CS required at time of application: Yes
including ECFMG Certificate
USCE Requirement: Yes 3 months
Cut-Off time since graduation: No limits set
Program offers couple match: Yes
Visas Sponsored or accepted: J1 visa

West Virginia

West Virginia University Combined Med-Peds Residency Program

Specialty: Combined Internal
Medicine/Pediatrics
Program name: West Virginia University
Program
Program code: 700-55-32-080
Program type: University-based
State: West Virginia
Address: West Virginia University School of
Medicine, Department of Pediatrics,
            PO Box 9214, Morgantown, WV
26506-9214
Phone: (304) 293-1224
Fax: (304) 293-1216

Percentage of IMGs in the program: 20%
Minimum USMLE Step 1 Score Requirement: 205
Minimum USMLE Step 2 Score Requirement: 205
Attempts on any step: No limits set
CS required at time of application: Yes
USCE Requirement: None
Cut-Off time since graduation: 5 years
Program offers couple match: Yes
Visas Sponsored or accepted: J1 visa

Marshall University School of Medicine Combined Med-Peds Residency Program

Specialty: Combined Internal Medicine/Pediatrics
Program name: Marshall University School of Medicine Program
Program code: 700-55-32-079
NRMP Code: 3066700C0
Program type: Community-based University affiliated hospital
State: West Virginia
Address: Marshall University School of Medicine, Suite 1039,
        1249 Fifteenth St, Huntington, WV 25701
Phone: (304) 691-1743

Fax: (304) 691-1745
Percentage of IMGs in the program: 0%
Minimum USMLE Step 1 Score Requirement:
No limits set
Minimum USMLE Step 2 Score Requirement:
No limits set
Attempts on any step: No limits set
CS required at time of application: Yes
including ECFMG certificate
USCE Requirement: None
Cut-Off time since graduation: 2 years
Program offers couple match: Yes
Visas Sponsored or accepted: J1 visa

Charleston Area Medical Center/West Virginia University (Charleston Division) Combined Med-Peds Residency Program

Specialty: Combined Internal
Medicine/Pediatrics
Program name: Charleston Area Medical
Center/West Virginia University (Charleston
Division) Program
Program code: 700-55-14-078
NRMP Code: 1902700C0
Program type: Community-based university
affiliated hospital
State: West Virginia

Address: Charleston Area Medical Center, Medicine/Pediatrics Program Ste 104,
830 Pennsylvania Ave, Charleston, WV 25302
Phone: (304) 388-1589
Fax: (304) 388-2926
Percentage of IMGs in the program: 25%
Minimum USMLE Step 1 Score Requirement: No limits set
Minimum USMLE Step 2 Score Requirement: No limits set
Attempts on any step: Must pass from first attempt
CS required at time of application: Yes including ECFMG certificate
USCE Requirement: None
Cut-Off time since graduation: No limits set
Program offers couple match: Yes
Visas Sponsored or accepted: J1 visa

Wisconsin

Medical College of Wisconsin Affiliated Hospitals Combined Med-Peds Residency Program

Specialty: Combined Internal Medicine/Pediatrics
Program name: Medical College of Wisconsin Affiliated Hospitals Program
Program code: 700-56-32-096
NRMP Code: 1784700C0
Program type: University-based
State: Wisconsin
Address: Children's Hospital Wisconsin, Children's Corporate Center Suite 430 PO 1997, 999 N 92nd St, Milwaukee, WI 53226
Phone: (414) 337-7030
Fax: (414) 337-7068
Percentage of IMGs in the program: 0%
Minimum USMLE Step 1 Score Requirement: No limits set
Minimum USMLE Step 2 Score Requirement: No limits set
Attempts on any step: No limits set
CS required at time of application: No
USCE Requirement: None
Cut-Off time since graduation: 5 years unless clinically active as in residency or practice
Program offers couple match: Yes
Visas Sponsored or accepted: J1 visa

Marshfield Clinic-St Joseph Hospital Combined Med-Peds Residency Program

Specialty: Combined Internal Medicine/Pediatrics
Program name: Marshfield Clinic-St Joseph's Hospital Program
Program code: 700-56-14-109
NRMP Code: 1780700C0
Program type: Community-based university affiliated hospital
State: Wisconsin
Address: Marshfield Clinic, Med-Peds Program 1F2,
      1000 N Oak Ave, Marshfield, WI 54449
Phone: (800) 541-2895   Ext: 93141
Fax: (715) 389-3142
Percentage of IMGs in the program: 60%
Minimum USMLE Step 1 Score Requirement: 210
Minimum USMLE Step 2 Score Requirement: 210
Attempts on any step: No limits set
CS required at time of application: Yes including ECFMG certificate
USCE Requirement: None
Cut-Off time since graduation: 5 years unless clinically active as in residency or practice
Program offers couple match: Yes
Visas Sponsored or accepted: J1 visa and H1b visa

I wish you good luck.

Thank you for buying our book.

Please, Please and Please take a minute to review our book on Amazon.

Match A Doc
Residency Guide

www.matchadoc.com